Breathing Meditations For Healing, Peace and Joy

Dr. Susan's Healthy Living
An imprint of Womens Wellness Publishing, LLC
drsusanshealthyliving.com

facebook.com/DrSusanLark
drsusanshealthyliving@gmail.com
(650) 561-9978

Mention of specific companies or products in this book does not suggest endorsement by the author or publisher. Internet addresses and telephone numbers for resources provided in this book were accurate at the time it went to press.

Cover design by Rebecca Rose

ISBN 978-1-939013-82-8

NOTE: The information in this book is meant to complement the advice and guidance of your physician, not replace it. It is very important that women who have medical problems should be evaluated by a physician. If you are under the care of a physician, you should discuss any major changes in your regimen with him or her. Because this is a book and not a medical consultation, keep in mind that the information presented here may not apply in your particular case. In view of individual medical requirements, new research, and government regulations, it is the responsibility of the reader to validate health practices and treatments with a physician or health service.

Acknowledgements

I want to give a huge thanks to my amazing editors Kendra Chun and Sandra K. Friend for their incredibly helpful assistance with putting this book together. I also greatly appreciate my fantastic Creative Director, Rebecca Richards, as well as Letitia Truslow, my wonderful Director of Media Relations. I enjoyed working with all of them and found their help indispensable in creating this exceptional book for women. Most of all, I want to thank God and Jesus Christ for their love and blessings.

Table of Contents

Part I:
Understanding Deep Breathing and Oxygenation

1

How Breathing and Oxygenation Benefit Your Health and Well-Being

The act of breathing is so vital to our health and well-being that it is mentioned in the Book of Genesis in the Judeo-Christian Bible, as our first connection with life. The Bible states "And the Lord God formed a man's body from the dust of the ground and breathed into it the breath of life. And the man became a living person."

I have always found this passage in the Bible to be fascinating and deeply moving. As a medical doctor, I am aware of how vital and precious many of our functions are — our brain is the seat of our intelligence, our heart pumps blood throughout our bodies and our kidneys are necessary to help remove waste products. But none of these important functions, except breathing, is highlighted and mentioned in the Bible as our first connection to life!

Take a deep breath right now and notice how good it feels. I always feel more alert, alive and refreshed when I pay attention to and focus on my breathing.

For years, I have observed people and their breathing patterns, including my patients, family members and friends and, of course, myself. I was fascinated to notice that the most healthy and vital people who seemed to radiate energy and joy of life were always deep breathers.

I also noticed that my patients who suffered from chronic lung problems, which affected their breathing capacity, seemed to be more tired, listless and devitalized than healthy breathers. Even stress and emotional upset causes our breathing to become more rapid and shallow, which cuts down on the amount of life giving oxygen we can take in from the air around us.

In fact, without healthy breathing, optimal health, wellness and enjoyment of life are virtually impossible.

This should be no surprise, since our lungs are responsible for interfacing with the air we breathe and flooding our bodies with life giving oxygen. Our bodies contain more oxygen than any other element.

Oxygen is an essential nutrient and a major component of our structure; it is fundamental to our very existence. Along with food, oxygen is the primary nutrient that cells use to generate energy for all their functions. Even a slight deficiency of oxygen in the cells can have a profound effect on our physical and mental performance as well as set the stage for the development of many diseases.

Because oxygen is so fundamental to our very existence, having sufficient levels within the body is a prerequisite for every aspect of health and peak performance. Sufficient oxygen is necessary for the energy and vitality, drive and determination, mental clarity, good social skills, and ability to recover from illness, injury, and exertion that are mandatory for a high level of performance in every area of life

I have included a detailed list of the benefits of the oxygen that we breathe in through our lungs in the following chart.

Benefits of Healthy Oxygenation

- Increased physical vitality and stamina (helps improve work productivity)

- Enhanced mental clarity and acuity

- Strengthened determination and perseverance in pursuing goals

- Increased ability to get along with other people (permits enjoyment of extensive social and business entertaining)

- Increased ability to remain calm under pressure

- Increased optimism and vision

- Increased resistance to illness

- Improves symptoms of skin conditions

- Promotes health of the teeth and gums

- Hastened recovery from illness, injury, and exertion (includes colds, flus, sinusitis, bronchitis, and allergies; athletic and repetitive-stress injuries; minor surgery; and dental procedures)

- Promotes healing and prevention of infectious diseases due to bacteria, viruses, and parasites

- Reduces the risk of cardiovascular disease

- Used as a complementary therapy for the treatment of cancer

- Helps in the treatment of gastrointestinal disorders

- Promotes healing of joint and bone diseases

- Helps in the treatment of neurological diseases such as multiple sclerosis

- Relieves cluster headaches

- Reverses age-related degeneration of vision

I wrote this book to share with you the program that I have developed to optimize breathing and oxygenation in the body. This program will help you to become healthier, stronger and more vital. The centerpiece of this book is twenty one wonderful breathing exercises that will promote healing, peace and joy as well as support your health and well-being. To provide additional health benefits to you, I have also included a guide on aerobic exercise, how to create a high oxygen content diet and information on nutrients that boost oxygenation and support lung health. I hope that you enjoy this program and find it to be valuable to improved health.

In the next three chapters, I share with you information about the chemistry of oxygenation, how oxygen is utilized in our bodies and how aging, lifestyle and health affect oxygenation.

You can either read these chapters to learn more about how breathing and oxygenation affect our health and wellness or you can skip these chapters and go on to Part II of this book to learn how to maintain healthy lungs and the therapies to optimize breathing and oxygenation in your body.

2

The Chemistry of Oxygenation

In this chapter, I share with you many interesting facts about the oxygen that we take into our bodies with every breath and the crucial role that it plays in our lives. The science of oxygen is fascinating since this important substance plays such a crucial role in our health and well-being.

Oxygen is the most abundant element on earth and is also the most important element needed to sustain life. It is a clear, odorless gas that easily dissolves in water. Because oxygen combines readily with other elements, it is the most abundant element on Earth, constituting about 50 percent of the weight of the Earth's crust, seawater, and atmosphere. Oxygen makes up approximately 20 percent of the composition of air by volume.

The body itself consists of four primary elements— hydrogen, nitrogen, oxygen, and carbon—which make up approximately 95 percent of the total mass of the body. Over two-thirds of this amount is oxygen. Each molecule of oxygen consists of two oxygen atoms and is described chemically as O_2.

Oxygen is the most important element needed to sustain life. Humans can survive without food for many weeks and can go without water for several days but can only survive without oxygen for a matter of minutes. We inhale between twelve to twenty times a minute while at rest, and much more frequently when we are engaged in strenuous physical activity. On average, we breathe in 2500 gallons of air every day.

Although oxygen is needed by all the cells and tissues of the body, much of the oxygen in the air we breathe is used by the heart, the liver, and especially the brain, which requires a disproportionate amount of oxygen. Even though the brain represents only about 2 percent of the weight of an average adult, it uses over 20 percent of the body's oxygen supply.

How Oxygen Is Taken into the Body

Oxygen is primarily taken into the body by the lungs during respiration. The lungs are two cone-shaped spongy organs. The wider part of the cone rests on the diaphragm just above the stomach. The left lung has an indentation to accommodate the heart, which sits slightly to the left between the two lungs. When we breathe, the lungs expand and contract like a bellows.

This continuously repeating movement also depends on the flexibility and movement of the various structures around the lungs. When we inhale, the diaphragm moves downward and the ribs elevate, increasing lung volume and capacity. When we exhale, the diaphragm automatically relaxes, the ribs lower, and the abdominal muscles contract. The lungs are then compressed, sending air out of the body.

When air is taken in through the mouth and nose, it moves toward the lungs. From the windpipe, air passes into two large bronchial tubes, which branch out into the bronchi and then into tiny bronchioles. Air finally enters the alveoli; these microscopic air sacs are the smallest compartments of the lung. There are 300 million alveoli in each lung. Because of this branching into smaller and smaller components, the lungs contain the equivalent of about 600 square feet of surface area. This enormous surface area allows for the efficient exchange of one of the body's primary waste products, carbon dioxide, for life-sustaining fresh oxygen.

Because of the structure of the alveoli, oxygen is able to diffuse into the blood. Although the walls of the alveoli are very thin, they contain a dense network of interconnecting capillaries, the smallest pathways through which blood circulates. Within the alveoli, oxygen from the air is now in close proximity to the capillaries and can enter the circulatory system. At this point, it is now considered to be inside the body, but the oxygen still has a long way to go before it reaches its final destination.

The circulatory system is made up of miles of capillaries and blood vessels that bring blood and oxygen to the tissues and cells throughout the body. When oxygen enters the body it first travels to the heart and then through these blood vessels. The veins collect waste products that accumulate in the cells, primarily carbon dioxide, which is generated in the production of energy. The veins bring the carbon dioxide back to the lungs. The carbon dioxide diffuses into the alveoli and then passes through ever-widening air passageways until it is exhaled.

Well-oxygenated blood in the arteries tends to be bright red, while the venous blood carrying all the waste products, especially carbon dioxide, tends to be darker. About 97 percent of the oxygen in the blood is carried in combination with hemoglobin, an iron-containing protein within the red blood cell. This allows oxygen to be delivered efficiently to all the cells of the body.

How Oxygen Is Used Within the Body

Oxygen is the primary fuel that supports all of the biochemical processes that occur in our tissues and cells. It supplies the energy for the maintenance, growth, and repair of our cells and tissues, and is crucial for maintaining our health and well-being at optimal levels.

The oxygen we breathe reacts with glucose (sugar), which is derived from the foods that we eat and from the breakdown of starches and fats in the body. This reaction produces carbon dioxide, water, and energy. The energy that is created from this reaction, which is a form of combustion, is stored in the body as adenosine triphosphate (ATP), which is often referred to as the basic energy currency of the body.

Because of its role in energy production, oxygen is essential for all of the tasks the cells must perform to maintain the health and integrity of the body, such as the transport of molecules, the synthesis of chemical compounds, and mechanical work like muscle contraction. Hundreds of thousands of these reactions are going on at all times.

Because of these reactions, the heart is able to pump blood, the immune system to fight infections, the gastrointestinal tract to digest foods, and the nervous system and brain to process information. Oxygen-generated energy is also fundamental to our ability to perform all physical movements.

Oxygen is an important structural component of the organic compounds used by the body as essential nutrients, such as vitamins, carbohydrates, and fatty acids. In addition, oxygen also has an important role in removing waste products from the body. When food is broken down and converted into energy, carbon residues can accumulate and must be removed from the body. This carbon combines with oxygen to form carbon dioxide, a waste product of metabolism that is excreted from the body through the lungs.

Oxygen is also alkaline and thereby helps the cells to maintain the slightly alkaline pH necessary for peak performance and optimal health. When a cell is highly oxygenated, it is able to create energy (ATP) through oxidative combustion, maintain its alkalinity, and sustain an environment that is incompatible with most disease-causing microorganisms.

However, when the amount of oxygen in the body is below optimal levels, this creates an environment in the cells that is conducive to the growth of infectious microorganisms. Most pathogens are anaerobic—that is, they thrive in an environment that is low in oxygen and has an acidic pH. In fact, infectious microorganisms such as bacteria, viruses, fungi, and parasites as well as cancer cells produce their energy (ATP) through the fermentation of glucose instead of through oxygen.

These pathogens are unable to survive in a cellular environment that is oxygen rich and slightly alkaline, which is why it is so critically important for peak performance and optimal health that we remain highly oxygenated and maintain our pH in a slightly alkaline state.

When a person becomes unable to fully oxygenate, an environment is created in which our energy begins to decline. We become fatigued, and disease and illness begin to occur with greater frequency. Over time, chronic conditions like heart disease and even cancer can develop. Finally, continued low levels of oxygenation increase the degenerative processes associated with aging and infirmity.

3

How Aging and Lifestyle Affect Oxygenation

If the body is not properly oxygenated through healthy breathing, the energy level within the body begins to decline, which can lead to fatigue, chronic illnesses, and degeneration. The next two chapters explain how aging, the way we live, and our health all affect our ability to oxygenate our bodies.

A wide variety of environmental and lifestyle factors, as well as certain diseases and the aging process itself, can cause oxygen levels in the body to decline. Outside of serious lung disease, blockage of the arteries, or anemia, no single factor alone can significantly reduce oxygen intake, but often a combination of factors can have a significant impact on a person's ability to maintain optimal oxygenation. For example, if a person does not exercise, is a moderate to heavy smoker, and develops a respiratory infection, then the ability to oxygenate can be seriously diminished, and the effects on performance and health can be significant. Very serious health conditions often develop from circumstances like these.

Aging

The cells of the body become damaged with age and cannot carry out their normal metabolic function, including the cell's ability to use oxygen. Damage to the cellular machinery occurs spontaneously during normal metabolism and also by contact with the large number of environmental pollutants and toxins to which people are exposed on a daily basis. These include heavy metals, pesticides, air pollution, outgassed toxins from indoor carpets and furniture, and a variety of other toxic agents with which people come in contact.

As people age, their lungs and cardiovascular systems become much less efficient in extracting oxygen from the air and delivering it to the cells. It also becomes more difficult for the cells to create energy through the metabolism of food and oxygen.

There are many reasons for this decline in function. Chronic muscle tension can become more of a problem as people age. This tension causes the muscles to lose their suppleness and flexibility, which restricts the action of the diaphragm and lungs. The aging process also brings about a loss of elasticity to all tissues, including the lungs. Much of the deterioration in breathing rate, lung capacity, and the ability to exchange gases is due to this loss. The rib cage, which expands and contracts with each breath, also becomes less elastic and pliable, and eventually the muscles in the lungs will weaken.

The very structure of the lungs changes over time, as airways narrow, the alveoli become flattened, and the alveolar ducts enlarge. All these factors contribute to a decrease in the ability of the body to take in oxygen. In addition, with age, cells throughout the body can become damaged simply from normal functioning and become less able to use the oxygen they receive.

Lifestyle

The air we breathe, the amount of stress we experience, and the food we eat all affect our oxygen levels. Our patterns of living, from our environment to our daily habits, are important indicators of the amount of oxygen we take in. Even the quality of the air we breathe can affect our oxygen levels.

Air pollution

It is estimated that over half the population of the United States regularly breathes unsafe, polluted air. Poor air quality is now commonplace in many of our leading cities, and many types of work expose people to unclean air that is dangerous to breathe.

For example, smog is a photochemical haze caused by the action of ultraviolet radiation on atmospheric pollution. It contains various toxins, including hydrocarbons and oxides of nitrogen from automobile exhaust. Nitrogen oxide is a primary industrial pollutant that reacts with sunlight and forms nitrogen dioxide, a brownish toxic gas.

A person may also be exposed to toxic airborne substances in the workplace, which can limit the ability of the lungs to provide the body with sufficient oxygen. Factory workers may be exposed to dust generated in the manufacture of certain products. Breathing dust composed of cotton, synthetic fibers, sugarcane, aluminum, or talc may be unavoidable. Workers in oil refineries may breathe sulfur dioxide, and people handling commercial refrigeration may be exposed to ammonia fumes. Servicing swimming pools exposes a person to chlorine-containing products, while health care professionals, roofers, woodworkers, welders, custodians, and firefighters often touch and handle toxic substances on a daily basis. Printers, lab workers, and painters breathe vapors from solvents and other toxic chemicals.

Our homes often contribute to the amount of airborne pollutants that we breathe in. Certain synthetic materials used in home furnishings such as carpets and upholstery can outgas—that is, they can emit volatile organic compounds such as toluene and xylene, known carcinogens such as formaldehyde and benzene, and pesticides that are toxic to our bodies. We also breathe fumes given off by cleaning agents, waxes, and polishes.

Office buildings, schools, stores, churches, and car interiors—any place that is furnished with products that outgas—can be a source of toxic substances. Another home pollutant is nitrogen oxide, which can originate from space heaters, unvented cooking stoves, and wood smoke.

When we inhale these toxic fumes and airborne pollutants, we breathe in less oxygen. In addition, these toxic substances can damage lung tissue and impair lung function, further limiting oxygen uptake. Normally, pollutants are blocked from entering the body as they pass through the upper airways of the respiratory system, the nose, sinuses, and throat. The upper airway cleans the air, clears it of particles, and inactivates microbes.

However, after heavy and/or prolonged exposure to air pollution, the system can become overwhelmed by toxins. At first, this may cause annoying symptoms such as inflammation, congestion, sneezing, and coughing similar to an allergic reaction. But if exposure persists, pollution can lead to lung damage. The lungs may become less flexible, and their ability to exchange carbon dioxide for oxygen may become impaired, causing the lungs and heart to work harder. Bronchitis and other chronic lung conditions may also develop.

Studies done in the past few years have examined the effects of pollution on the health of people living in cities with heavy levels of air pollution. For example, several studies have examined air quality and its impact on the health of people in Mexico City, where air pollution can far surpass acceptable levels. Residents of Mexico City showed significantly more signs of lung damage than people living in unpolluted cities in Mexico. In addition, even visitors suffered from respiratory irritation when exposed to high levels of smog-ridden air. These changes persisted even after the visitors had returned home, abating only several weeks later.

Many people living in cities make a special effort to exercise outdoors to bolster their health and well-being. However, if exercise is performed on smoggy days or near highways, this well-intentioned physical activity may often do more harm than good. When a person does vigorous exercise, they breathe through the mouth, and air does not pass through the nose to be cleaned. A person jogging in smog will inhale dirty air deep into their lungs, where it can affect the health of the lungs and oxygen intake.

Smoking

One particularly lethal form of air pollution is cigarette smoke, whether a person smokes and inhales the toxins directly or inhales it secondhand from someone else's cigarette. Smoking limits the amount of oxygen that reaches our cells and tissues in several ways.

Cigarette smoke irritates lung tissue, particularly the cilia. Cilia are threadlike projections that line the respiratory passages and normally sweep back and forth, moving debris out of the lungs. Cigarette smoke paralyzes the cilia, especially the smoke from menthol cigarettes. In response, the lungs produce mucus, which covers the cilia and further prevents them from doing their job of cleaning. As debris accumulates, the alveoli become damaged, impairing the uptake of oxygen into the circulation.

Cigarette smoke also decreases the amount of hemoglobin in the blood. As a result, the blood cannot carry as much oxygen to the cells. Smoking can also lead to health problems that are associated with low levels of oxygen such as respiratory infections, pneumonia, chronic bronchitis, and lung cancer. These diseases, in turn, often damage the lungs, which further impairs oxygen uptake.

Carbon monoxide

Carbon monoxide is formed by the combustion of carbon in oxygen when there is an excess of carbon. It is generated in coal stoves, furnaces, and gas appliances that do not get enough air. It is also present in the exhaust of automobiles. Early symptoms of carbon monoxide poisoning include headaches and drowsiness, followed by unconsciousness, respiratory failure, and death.

Carbon monoxide can be a particularly lethal component of air in that it has no odor, so a person isn't aware of inhaling it. According to an article published in the *Journal of the American Medical Association*, there are approximately 2100 deaths from carbon monoxide poisoning in the United States each year. Hemoglobin (the oxygen-carrying protein in red blood cells) has a much greater affinity for carbon monoxide than oxygen.

As carbon monoxide in the air we breathe is only a very recent phenolmenon, the body is not designed to block it from entering the system. In the alveoli of the lungs, where gases from the outside are exchanged with gases from within the body, hemoglobin, which usually carries molecules of oxygen through the body, is over two hundred times as likely to grab onto a molecule of carbon monoxide instead. Therefore, any exposure to carbon monoxide limits the amount of oxygen uptake as well as the quantity reaching the cells.

Stress

Being caught in a seemingly unending traffic jam or spending the day hunched over a computer trying to finish a late report causes physical and emotional stress that can affect breathing by causing our muscles to tighten. Stress also causes breathing to become rapid and shallow. A person may even stop breathing altogether and hold their breath for brief periods without realizing it.

All of these changes in breathing patterns cause less oxygen to be taken in through respiration, which decreases the oxygen available to the muscles and internal organs. Under stress, a person will also tense muscles in certain parts of the body, commonly the shoulders and neck, involuntarily preparing for a fight as the automatic stress response sets in. Blood vessels also constrict, reducing circulation to the tense muscles and preventing oxygen from reaching these areas and carbon dioxide from being eliminated.

If a person leads a life in which nearly every day is stressful, such muscle tension can become chronic. Over time, this constant tension reduces the amount of oxygen that reaches the cells, and performance and health begin to suffer as a result.

Lack of aerobic exercise

A sedentary lifestyle can weaken the lungs, heart, and blood vessels, reducing the amount of oxygen taken into the body and transported to the tissues. Lack of exercise reduces the efficiency of lung function. The lungs are not able to fully expand and fill with air. The heart will not pump as forcefully to circulate blood and oxygen throughout the body. One benefit of physical activity is to dilate (expand) the network of blood vessels so blood reaches the muscles and vital organs as well as the small capillaries. When a person does not exercise, this expansion of the circulatory system is diminished.

Techniques for retaining physical flexibility, such as stretching and yoga, can serve several purposes. By promoting muscular flexibility, these techniques significantly enhance the mechanics of breathing, thereby assisting the flow of oxygen to the cells and the removal of carbon dioxide. These slow, methodical exercises also reduce muscle tension. As you relax, the other effects of stress are gradually reduced. Also, stretching exercises and yoga can be practiced almost anywhere, which is a great benefit to travelers.

Diet

Foods that are highest in water content, such as raw vegetables and fruit, are also highest in their oxygen content. Remember that water is the most abundant substance on the earth's surface and that most of our bodies consist of water and, thereby, oxygen. Thus, a diet that contains plenty of fresh, raw vegetables and fruit can significantly contribute to our supply of oxygen.

Unfortunately, processed and refined foods usually have a much lower water content than the original fresh ingredients. This can even be true of frozen foods, such as strawberries: Once defrosted, they lose most of their water content. Also, the foods that make up the standard American diet are highly processed and refined. These foods tend to be highly acidic, further reducing the stores of oxygen within the body.

4

Health Conditions that Limit Oxygenation

A number of diseases limit how much oxygen is taken into the body. These include a wide variety of conditions, including some lung diseases such as asthma, bronchitis, and pneumonia. Whatever the cause of the damage to the lung, the end result is the same: The lungs are less able to breathe in oxygen and transfer it to the blood for circulation throughout the body. Atherosclerosis, anemia, and chronic-fatigue syndrome also affect the amount of oxygen in the body.

In extreme cases, patients with severe respiratory diseases may end up in the hospital on assisted breathing. I have worked with many patients in the hospital whose ability to breathe was compromised by severe lung disease and who were only able to survive thanks to the use of ventilators.

I have seen teenagers and young adults who were on ventilators because of extremely severe asthmatic attacks or morbid obesity as well as middle aged or elderly persons suffering from pneumonia or severe chronic lung disease. Everyone with compromised breathing who regains his or her ability to breathe in a healthy manner is truly relieved and grateful.

Health issues that can affect the ability to breathe or take in and distribute oxygen from the environment include the following:

Sinusitis

The term sinusitis refers to an infection lodged in any of the four sacs of air cells that surround both sides of the nose. Sinuses have openings into the nose that are quite small and easily blocked by thick secretions and swelling. When blockage occurs, the warm, moist environment within the sinuses is a ready breeding ground for bacteria. As a result, breathing becomes more difficult.

Chronic bronchitis

Shallow breathing can also occur with chronic bronchitis. This ailment involves persistent inflammation of the air passageways within the lungs. It is often characterized by the excessive secretion of mucous and a chronic cough. Smokers are at higher risk of developing this condition.

Emphysema

In this disease, the alveoli are destroyed; impairing the exchange of oxygen and carbon dioxide, and oxygen does not as readily diffuse into the blood. The lungs enlarge, but they work less efficiently, often painfully and with great effort.

Asthma

Asthma is usually due to an allergic reaction to a substance such as pollen. It can also be triggered, in some individuals, by strong emotions. When a person has an asthmatic attack, tissues in the passageways of the lungs swell and become narrower. The muscles involved in breathing may contract. Exhaling can become very difficult, and the proper exchange of oxygen and carbon dioxide is prevented.

Pneumonia

Pneumonia is an infectious disease in which the alveoli become infected with bacteria. The membranes within the alveoli become inflamed and porous. The alveoli become filled with fluids and blood cells. Symptoms of pneumonia can include coughing, sputum production, and a high fever.

Tuberculosis

In recent years, there has been an increase in the incidence of tuberculosis, a potentially dangerous bacterial disease, especially in inner cities. In tuberculosis, fibrous tissue usually forms to wall off the infected area. This is the body's way of limiting the spread of the disease. However, in about 3 percent of cases, this process fails, and the disease spreads throughout the lungs. This reduces the total amount of functional lung tissue, limiting the amount of oxygen the lungs can hold and the amount of oxygen that diffuses into the blood.

Atherosclerosis

The circulatory system consists of miles of arteries and capillaries that bring oxygen to the tissues. Anything that causes a narrowing or occlusion of these blood vessels can affect oxygenation. Plaque, an accumulation of cholesterol and fibrous tissue on the arterial walls, is one of the most common causes of such narrowing. The buildup of plaque is often referred to as "hardening of the arteries," or atherosclerosis.

The plaque may accumulate sufficiently in certain places to decrease blood flow and obstruct circulation. In these areas, oxygenation and the flow of nutrients to the tissue can be drastically reduced. Hypertension (high blood pressure) can also limit oxygenation since it causes the blood vessels to contract. This forces the heart to work harder to move the same amount of blood to the tissues.

Anemia

It is estimated that as many as 20 percent of all American women suffer from anemia, which is a deficiency of red blood cells or a reduction in hemoglobin (the oxygen-carrying protein in red blood cells). Anemia may be due to blood loss, diminished blood production, a failure of the red blood cells to mature because of a lack of vitamin B12 or folic acid, or hemolysis, in which the red blood cells break apart.

Anemia reduces the amount of oxygen available to all cells of the body. As a result, less oxygen is available for energy production by the cells. Important processes such as muscular activity and cell building and repair slow down and become less efficient. As a result, anemia can be debilitating and result in profound physical fatigue.

Because of this reduction in blood cells, individuals who are anemic tend to be pale with poor skin color and tone. They often appear washed-out and seem listless. Individuals with anemia usually feel extremely fatigued. Because muscular activity is inhibited, those suffering from anemia lack endurance and physical stamina.

I have had had many physically active patients who had to stop pursuing vigorous aerobic exercise programs when they developed anemia. These people simply lacked the physical energy to continue their active exercise regimens once the anemia became too severe. Many people who are chronically tired are suffering from a low-grade anemia that needs to be treated.

Chronic-Fatigue Syndrome

Chronic fatigue syndrome (CFS), a condition in which fatigue is debilitating if not incapacitating, has been diagnosed in over 3 million Americans. The onset of fatigue is often sudden; many individuals can pinpoint exactly when it started. The fatigue is so severe that even minor exertion, such as a short walk or light housework, can be difficult to accomplish. Many people with CFS curtail their activities and take naps during the day, or sleep more hours at night. However, increased bed rest does not improve the energy level of those with this problem. Their breathing may be weak and shallow.

The most widely accepted hypothesis is that CFS is due to a viral infection, although this has not been definitely proven. Most of the attention has focused on the herpes family of viruses, such as Epstein-Barr virus. In addition, though, people who have CFS tend to be poorly oxygenated. Patients may indeed be infected by a virus, but viruses thrive in oxygen-depleted environments.

A wide variety of environmental and lifestyle factors may also contribute to CFS by stressing the immune system. Many of my CFS patients report extreme and prolonged emotional stress, anxiety, and depression, and a history of poor nutritional habits predating the onset of CFS. Environmental pollutants and contaminants may also play a role in weakening the body and allowing CFS to develop. All these related conditions further reduce oxygen within the body.

5

How Healthy Are Your Breathing and Oxygenation Checklists

To learn whether you are breathing deeply and efficiently and if your ability to oxygenate your body can support optimal health and wellness, I suggest that you work through the following checklists. You can copy them if you don't want to write in the book. You can then refer to the checklists as you read through the rest of the book. Doing so will help you to assess how healthy your breathing capacity is and how well your body is oxygenated.

Putting a check mark beside any of the items listed could mean that your breathing is shallow or impaired, your lungs are being stressed or that your body is not receiving sufficient oxygen.

If you find that a number of the statements in the checklist apply to you, you should implement a program to improve your breathing and restore your oxygen levels. Your responses to this checklist can also help you decide whether you need to exercise more, change your diet, or make a more conscious effort to breathe deeply. You may also realize that your environment needs upgrading to provide you with better-quality air to breathe or water to drink. As always, consult a health care professional if you think that you may have a serious health condition.

Lifestyle/Environmental Factors

Put a check mark beside those statements that are true for you.

- I rarely eat fresh fruits and vegetables.

- I eat mostly overcooked foods and foods that are processed.

- I smoke cigarettes.

- I walk or exercise along streets filled with traffic.

- I lead a sedentary lifestyle.

- I tend to stand and move with a stiff, military posture.

- I habitually feel stressed and uptight.

- I regularly spend long hours engaged in desk work.

- I spend much of every day working at a computer.

- I live in a major metropolitan area.

- My home is in a city with a smog problem.

- I recently moved into a new house or apartment.

- My floors are covered with carpets made of synthetic fibers.

- I regularly burn wood in the fireplace.

- I cook on an unvented stove.

- I work in a building that has sealed windows.

- My profession involves exposure to chemical toxins (for example, I am a painter, firefighter, hairstylist, or health care worker or I work in a dry-cleaning establishment).

- I work in a factory where there is dust from cotton, synthetic fibers, sugarcane, aluminum, or talc. I work in an oil refinery or in a plant that produces or utilizes toxic chemicals.

Performance indicators

- I have little energy for recreational activities or spending time with family and friends.

- I rarely participate in meetings and have difficulty coming up with new ideas.

- I often have difficulty concentrating.

- I am often unable to remember names.

- I am frequently unable to see a project through to completion.

- I lack goals and inspiration.

- I am slow to recover from injury, illness, and physical exertion.

- I have limited stamina and endurance while exercising.

- I am easily fatigued and usually tired at the end of the-day.

- I find myself out of breath after running for the phone.

- I am out of breath after climbing a flight of stairs.

- I lack close social and personal relationships.

- I am introverted and don't enjoy social gatherings.

- I am generally pessimistic.

Medical history

- I have frequent episodes of colds, flus, bronchitis, pneumonia, allergies, or sinusitis.

- I tend to be anemic.

- I have a history of emphysema, chronic bronchitis, lung infections, or asthma.

- I suffer from cardiovascular or vascular disease.

- I suffer from chronic-fatigue syndrome.

Now that you have a preliminary understanding of the importance of oxygenation to optimal health and wellness, as well as some idea from the checklist of your own functioning in this area, you can learn how to support healthy breathing and oxygenation in the following chapters.

In Part II of this book, I share with you how to support the health of your lungs and restore your oxygen levels through breathing exercises, aerobic exercise, nutritional supplementation and an oxygen rich diet.

Part II:
Supporting Healthy Breathing and Oxygenation

6

Breathing Exercises for Health and Wellness

In this chapter, I share with you breathing exercises that I have developed to help restore healthy breathing and oxygenation. I recommend that you try all of the exercises in this chapter, and then practice the ones you like the most on a regular basis. Many of my patients have practiced these deep breathing exercises along with other stress reduction techniques and have found them to be very helpful.

Perform these exercises in a slow and relaxed manner. Breathing slowly and deeply allows you take in large amounts of oxygen from the environmental air. Full expansion of the lungs in a relaxed, rhythmic way facilitates maximal oxygen uptake by the body. It is important to allow both the stomach and the rib cage to relax while breathing so that air can fill the entire lungs. This type of breathing strengthens the muscles in the abdomen and chest, relaxes the body, and allows for the most efficient oxygenation.

Practicing these breathing exercises on a regular basis is a wonderful antidote to stress. Often, our busy stress filled lives make deep, healthy breathing more difficult. When you are stressed or tense, breathing becomes more erratic and shallow. As a result, your oxygen levels will decrease. You may find yourself breathing too fast, or you may even stop breathing altogether and hold your breath for prolonged periods of time without realizing it. If you catch yourself doing this, it is very beneficial to stop what you are doing and take a "breath break." Taking time each day to relax for a few minutes and do breathing exercises can reverse this pattern of stress and help restore a sense of peace and calm to your life.

Therapeutic breathing exercises are also a simple, yet powerful way, to relieve pain and discomfort in your body. When you are feeling pain, breathing tends to become jagged, erratic, and shallow and your oxygen levels decrease. As with stress and anxiety, you tend to tense and tighten your muscles, constrict blood flow, elevate your pulse rate and heartbeat, and stimulate the output of stressful chemicals from your glands as a response to the pelvic discomfort. Waste products such as carbon dioxide and lactic acid also accumulate in your muscles and other tissues.

Practicing breathing exercises provides a way to break up this pattern of stress and help the body return to equilibrium. This process gives you more voluntary control over managing your discomfort. Through the use of controlled breathing exercises, you can relax and loosen your muscles, decrease sensations of pain, lower your anxiety level, and generate a feeling of internal peace and calm.

Finally, breathing exercises are a great way to reduce tiredness and fatigue and create more energy and vitality in every cell of your body. Therapeutic breathing is of major benefit to women suffering from chronic fatigue. Women who are tired tend to restrict their movements in general. They exercise less, go out socially less frequently, and even restrict their household tasks. They spend more time lying on the bed or couch.

When movement is limited in this way, breathing tends to become shallow and restricted. Instead of the deep abdominal breathing that we see with healthy aerobic activity, fatigued women may find that they practically stop breathing altogether and hold their breath for prolonged periods of time without even realizing it. The end result is a decrease in oxygen levels in the body, poorer blood circulation, muscle tension, and a decrease in metabolic activity of the cells.

It is important to do the breathing exercises in this chapter in a slow and relaxed manner. You can do them in a bright and cheerful part of your home or even outdoors in your backyard or in a park. When you begin your breathing exercise session, it is important to find a comfortable position. You should do some exercises lying on your back; for other exercises, you'll be sitting up. Unless otherwise directed, keep your arms and legs uncrossed and your back straight.

Exercise 1: Deep Abdominal Breathing

Deep, slow abdominal breathing is a very important technique to optimize our intake of oxygen, increase our level of energy and bring us a sense of deep inner peace, calm and joy. It helps brings more oxygen, the fuel for metabolic activity, to all tissues of the body. Rapid, shallow breathing decreases oxygen supply and keeps one devitalized. Deep breathing helps to relax the entire body, and strengthens muscles in the chest and abdomen. It also helps calm many other physiological processes, such as rapid pulse rate and heartbeat that often accompany stress and pain.

- Lie flat on your back with your knees pulled up. Keep your feet slightly apart. Try to breathe in and out through your nose.

- Inhale deeply. As you breathe in, allow your stomach to relax so that the air flows into your abdomen. Your stomach should balloon out as you breathe in. Visualize your lungs filling up with air so that your chest swells out.

- Imagine that the air you breathe is filling your body with energy.

- Exhale deeply. As you breathe out, let your stomach and chest collapse. Imagine the air being pushed out, first from your abdomen and then from your lungs.

Exercise 2: Peaceful, Slow Breathing

Breathing slowly and peacefully can actually decrease anxiety and help to promote a sense of inner calm and quiet. Such breathing helps our mind to slow down and our emotions to be happier and more harmonious. Life feels good. We make better decisions and relate to those around us in a healthier way when we are calm. Breathing slowly can calm our physical responses by helping to balance autonomic nervous system function. The autonomic nervous system regulates functions that we're usually not aware of, such as circulation of the blood, muscle tension, pulse rate, breathing, and glandular function.

The autonomic nervous system is divided into two parts that oppose and complement each other, the sympathetic and parasympathetic systems. The sympathetic nervous system is linked to tension and the "fight or flight" response of fear and panic, while the parasympathetic nervous system regulates body responses that are relaxed and calm. Slow, peaceful breathing is a way to calm down these stress responses and bring the body back to a state of balance. By slowing down our breathing, we slow down our other physiologic responses. Our muscles relax and our blood vessels dilate; a state of equilibrium is restored.

- Lie flat on your back with your knees pulled up. Keep your feet slightly apart. Try to breathe in and out through your nose.

- Inhale deeply. As you breathe in, allow your stomach to relax so that the air flows into your abdomen. Let your stomach balloon out as you breathe in. Visualize the lowest parts of your lungs filling up with air.

- Imagine that the air you are breathing in is filled with peace and calm. A sensation of peacefulness and calm is filling every cell of your body. Your whole body feels warm and relaxed as you breathe in this air. Now, exhale deeply. As you breathe out, imagine the air being pushed out from the bottom of your lungs to the top.

- Repeat this sequence until your entire body feels relaxed and your breathing is slow and regular.

Exercise 3: Grounding

When women are experiencing pain and discomfort, they often lose a sense of being grounded, literally rooted to the earth. Some women report a sensation of numbness in their legs and feet. They may say that they feel as if they have no legs at all. Pelvic and low back pain causes leg muscles to tighten and decrease blood circulation and oxygenation to lower extremities. This physical response to pain is part of the reason we lose the sense of owning our legs. When we are physically ungrounded, it is very difficult to function mentally; we have a hard time focusing and concentrating. When our bodies are uncomfortable, we may have difficulty working through our projects for the day in a coherent manner.

Sit upright in a chair. Be sure you are in a comfortable position. Keep your feet slightly apart. Breathe in and out through your nose.

- Inhale deeply. As you breathe in, allow your stomach to relax so that the air flows into your abdomen. Let your stomach balloon out as you breathe in. Visualize the lowest parts of your lungs filling up with air. Hold your inhalation.

- Visualize a golden cord with a golden ball at the end of it running from the base of your spine. Let this golden cord gently and slowly move downwards through the earth, grounding you. You can let it move down as far as you would like, even all the way to the center of the earth.

- Follow the cord and its golden ball in your mind all the way down and see it fasten securely to the earth's center. You can run two golden cords from the bottoms of your feet down to the center of the earth, also, if you would like.

- As you exhale, become aware of your hips, thighs, calves, ankles, and feet. Feel their strength and solidity.

- Repeat this exercise several times until you feel fully present and grounded.

Exercise 4: Muscle Tension Release Breathing

This exercise will help you to get in touch with and release general muscle tension and tightness. Often we carry extra tension in our bodies when we are feeling stressed, driving in rush hour traffic, dealing with upset children, doing intense desk work or even competitive sports. These are typical of activities that may cause us to tense our muscles and breathe less deeply. We may unconsciously tense up muscles throughout the entire body. Doing intense work at the computer frequently creates tension in the neck, shoulders and not even be aware of it.

I want to share with you a wonderful exercise that will help you to get in touch with and release any muscle tension and tightness and bring your body back into a state of healthy balance. Often when you are stressed anxious and upset, you may unconsciously tense up muscles throughout the entire body. The neck, shoulders, lower back, hips and other areas of the body are particularly vulnerable.

Muscle tension often occurs in response to the stresses of the day or from sitting in one position for hours at the desk or computer and even after doing vigorous exercise. After doing this meditation, you will feel more peaceful and relaxed!

- Sit or lie in a comfortable position. Allow your arms to rest at your sides, palms down and inhale and exhale slowly and deeply.

- Become aware of your feet, ankles, and legs. Notice if these parts of your body have any muscle tension or tightness. Breathe into that part of your body until you feel it relax.

- Next, move your awareness into your hips, pelvis, and lower back. Note any tension there. Breathe into your hips and pelvis until you feel them relax. Release any emotional stress as you breathe in and out.

- Focus on your abdomen and chest. Notice any tension or tightness located in this area and let it drop away as you breathe in and out. Continue to breathe into this area until your chest and abdomen feel relaxed.

- Finally, focus on your head, neck, arms, and hands. Note any tension in this area and release it. With your breathing, release any negative emotions blocked in this area until you feel peaceful and calm.

- When you have finished releasing tension throughout the body, continue deep breathing and relaxing for another minute or two. At the end of this exercise, you should feel lighter, relaxed and more energized.

Exercise 5: Breathing to Release Tension in the Upper Body

This exercise will help you focus on any tension that you are carrying in your upper body. As you relax and release the muscles in your neck and shoulders, it will help to release muscle tension in your entire body. This is a good exercise to do while walking or doing sports or desk work, to get in touch with any muscle tension that you may be carrying.

- Sit upright in a chair. Be sure you are in a comfortable position. Keep your feet slightly apart. Try to breathe in and out through your nose.

- Inhale and exhale deeply. As you breathe, let your head move from side to side, keeping your shoulders down. As you do this movement, imagine that your neck is made out of putty and that it allows your head to move in a supple, relaxed movement from the left to the right.

- Now inhale and pull your shoulders up towards your ears.

- Hold your breath and keep your shoulders in a hunched position. Exhale and let your shoulders drop back into a relaxed, comfortable position. Repeat this several times.

- Inhale and exhale deeply as you roll your shoulders forward. Make a large, slow, circular motion with your shoulders. Then, roll your shoulders back slowly. Repeat this several times.

- Inhale and exhale deeply, keeping the rest of your body still and relaxed. Repeat this several times.

Exercise 6: Emotional Cleansing Breath

I have seen, during my years of medical practice, that muscle tension and pain is worse when women are under emotional stress. The more day-to-day stress that you have, related to family, work, and other personal issues, the more you may experience increased muscle tension and pain. Many of my patients have told me that their unhealed family and other personal relations, as well as sexual problems, are also significant emotional triggers for their sensations of pain and discomfort.

This exercise uses breathing to help you release any negative feelings, such as chronic anger or upset that you may be harboring. The more time you spend cleansing old negative emotional patterns, the less these feelings can create pain and tension in your body.

Lie flat on your back with your knees pulled up. Keep your feet slightly apart. Try to breathe in and out through your nose.

- Inhale deeply and see yourself enveloped in a soft white light. Breathe this light into every cell of your body. This is a cleansing light and can help wash away fear, anger, anxiety, and other negative feelings.

- As you exhale deeply, feel the light washing these emotions away.

- Repeat this exercise until you feel emotionally peaceful and clear.

Exercise 7: Color Breathing with Red

Color breathing has traditionally been used to strengthen the body's energy field and heal the body. Intuitives can see this energy field as light or colors emanating from the body. When a person is calm, relaxed, and healthy, the energy field appears radiant and full of colors. The colors are bright and harmonious, and each one corresponds to specific parts of the body.

When we are feeling pain or tension, we lose our light and color. Our energy field looks more discordant and jagged, and often the colors change in response to the physical discomfort to duller, more muddied colors.

Color breathing is a technique that can help strengthen and heal the energy field as well as the body itself. As you breathe in the healing color, the parts of your body that are in pain and discomfort often begin to relax and feel healthier again. Tension and cramping is replaced by a sensation of lightness and peace.

- Sit or lie in a comfortable position.

- Take a deep breath and visualize that the earth below you is filled with a bright red color. Imagine that you are opening up energy centers on the bottom of your feet. See this color flowing into your feet as you inhale; visualize the bright red color filling up your feet.

- Draw this color up your legs and into your lower body. See it first filling up your legs, then your lower back, and finally your pelvis. Your lower body is filling with a beautiful bright red color. As you exhale, see this color flow out of your lower body and fill the air around you. Exhale the bright red slowly out of your lungs.

- Next, as you inhale deeply, continue to draw the bright red color into your abdomen, chest, arms, neck and head. As you exhale, see this color flow out of your upper body and fill the air around you. Exhale the bright red slowly out of your lungs.

Exercise 8: Color Breathing with Blue

In this exercise, the color sky blue is used to promote peace, calm, and relaxation. It also helps to relax tense and tight muscles. This is a very helpful exercise to do if you are feeling stressed and anxious because it has a calming effect on the brain and nervous system.

- Take a deep breath and visualize that the earth below you is filled with a sky blue color. See this color flowing into your feet as you inhale; visualize the sky blue color filling up your feet.

- Draw this color up your legs and into your lower body. See it first filling up your legs, then your lower back, and finally your pelvis. Your lower body is filling with a beautiful sky blue color. As you exhale, see this color flow out of your lower body and fill the air around you. Exhale the sky blue slowly out of your lungs.

- Next, as you inhale deeply, continue to draw the sky blue color into your abdomen, chest, arms, neck and head. As you exhale, see this color flow out of your upper body and fill the air around you. Exhale the sky blue slowly out of your lungs.

Exercise 9: Color Breathing with Golden Light

- Sit or lie in a comfortable position.

- Imagine a cloud of beautiful golden energy surrounding you. As you take a deep breath, inhale the golden energy and visualize it flowing through your body, into your feet, legs hips and lower back. Then loving into your abdomen, chest, arms, neck and head. This is a healing energy—it warms and relaxes you're your entire body, bringing you back into a state of health and balance. Hold the inhalation as long as it is comfortable. Let this golden cloud pick up all your pain and tension.

- Then exhale this energy out through your lungs and be carried away from you.

- Repeat this process as many times as you need to, until the pain is replaced by a feeling of peace and calm.

Exercise 10: Energy Breathing for the Entire Body

This breathing exercise combines imagery with deep breathing. As you visualize the energizing effects that breathing has on your body, you actually begin to lay down a mental blueprint for enhanced health and well-being.

This exercise promotes energy and vitality by directing your breath into every part of your body. This helps release stress and muscle tension in parts of your body that you aren't even aware is tense; it elevates the energy of the whole body. It reinforces the importance of the body functioning as a whole, integrated unit for optimal health and well-being. This exercise should leave you with a greater degree of energy and vitality as well as deeply peaceful and calm.

- Lie flat on your back with your knees pulled up. Keep your feet slightly apart. Breathe in and out through your nose, if possible.

- Inhale deeply. As you breathe in, allow your stomach to relax so that the air flows into your abdomen. Let your stomach balloon out as you breathe in. Visualize the lowest parts of your lungs filling up with air. Then exhale deeply. As you breathe out, imagine the air being pushed out from the bottom of your lungs to the top.

- Now visualize that the air you are breathing is filled with energy and vitality. Let this energy flow into your feet, legs, hips, pelvis and then into your abdomen, chest, arms, neck and head. Feel a renewed sense of vitality filling every cell of your body. It fills you with a sensation of warmth and healing.

- Now, exhale deeply. As you breathe out, imagine the air being pushed out from the bottom of your lungs to the top.

- Repeat this sequence until your entire body feels relaxed and your breathing is slow and regular.

Exercise 11: Hara Breathing

In Chinese healing, the hara is one of the most important centers of vitality. In fact, it is called the "Sea of Energy." The hara point, located three finger-widths below the naval, is considered the center of the body in traditional Chinese healing models.

Stimulation of the hara point helps to strengthen the body, as well as improve energy and endurance. Hara breathing nourishes and energizes the internal organs, improving health in general as well as helping to relieve chronic fatigue and tiredness.

- Sit upright in a chair, with your arms at your sides. First, find the hara point with your fingers. Then, as you inhale deeply, draw breath into your lower abdomen and focus on concentrating your breath into the hara point. Feel the hara point expand and energize.

- As you exhale, feel the hara point and your lower abdomen release the life energy so that it circulates throughout your body.

- Repeat this exercise for several minutes—drawing breath and energy into the hara point as you inhale, then circulating life energy throughout your body as you exhale.

Exercise 12: Breath of Fire

This short, rapid breathing technique is used in stretches to charge the body with immediate energy. This exercise also energizes the nervous system and stimulates blood circulation.

•   Sit upright in a chair, your arms at your sides, palms up. As you inhale, fill your abdomen with a deep breath. Then breathe rapidly out through your nose, exhaling one short breath every second or two. As you breathe out, contract your abdomen by pumping in and out until your lungs are empty.

•   Repeat several times until you feel energized and fully awake and present.

Exercise 13: Glandular Breathing

Your endocrine glands support female hormonal health, mental clarity and many essential functions to optimize health. This exercise helps stimulate and energize your endocrine glands through the use of color breathing. When you direct your breath into the endocrine glands and visualize them being stimulated by the color, the glands are, in fact, stimulated in a beneficial way. The use of color breathing expands the electromagnetic field of the endocrine glands. In this exercise, the color red is used; in research studies, red light has been shown to stimulate both the endocrine and immune functions.

- Sit upright in a chair, your arms at your sides, palms up. Visualize a soft cloud or energy field filled with the color red above your head. It is a bright, vibrant tone of red that sparkles with energy.

- As you inhale deeply, see the red energy flowing into your head and concentrating in the hypothalamus. You can visualize the area of this endocrine gland by focusing the red energy in the area between your eyes (sometimes called "the third eye" area). As the hypothalamus begins to overflow with color, exhale and let the red energy flow out of your lungs, filling the air around you.

- As you inhale again, breathe the bright red color into your pituitary, an important endocrine gland located in your brain, right below the hypothalamus. Fill the pituitary with this color until it overflows. Then exhale deeply releasing any excess red energy.

- As you continue to inhale the bright red color, let it flow into your thyroid gland, located at the base of your neck, then into your thymus gland, located in the middle of your chest. Finally, let the color energize your adrenal glands, located in the middle of your back above the kidneys, and finally your pelvis. As you fill up each endocrine gland with red energy, continue to release any excess energy into the air around you as you exhale.

- When you finish this exercise, relax for a few minutes. You should feel energized and bright, yet peaceful and calm at the same time.

Exercise 14: Depression Release Breathing

Depression often accompanies chronic fatigue and tiredness. When a woman is tired, often her mood is low, too. It is hard to feel enthusiastic and high-spirited about life when you have no energy and vitality supporting your mental processes. This next exercise helps to elevate mood and enhance emotional well-being through focused breathing.

- Sit upright in a chair. Your arms are crossed in front of your chest with your fingers touching the upper outer area of your chest. Your wrist crosses over your heart chakra, which is the energy center for emotions and feelings.

- As you inhale, imagine a golden light filling your heart center with a warm, loving feeling. As you exhale, breathe out depression and low spirits.

- As you inhale again, draw this golden light up through your neck and into your head. See it illuminating your head with a soft, peaceful glow. Feel any depression or negative thoughts dissolving as the golden light fills every cell in your brain.

- As you exhale, breathe the golden light out through the top of your head and see it form a shimmering cloud of energy around your entire body.

- Repeat the exercise 5 times.

Exercise 15: Emotional Healing Breath

During my years of medical practice, I have found that emotional stress is a significant trigger for fatigue and exhaustion. Holding emotional upset literally drains our energy. This exercise uses breathing to help you release negative feelings such as chronic anger, hurt, or other upsets you may be harboring. The more time you spend cleansing old negative emotional patterns, the less impact these feelings will have on your energy level.

- Lie flat on your back with your knees pulled up. Keep your feet slightly apart. Try to breathe in and out through your nose.

- Inhale deeply and see yourself enveloped in a soft white light.

- Breathe this light into every cell of your body. This is a cleansing light and can help wash away fear, anger, anxiety, and other negative feelings.

- As you exhale deeply, feel the light washing these emotions away.

- Continue to repeat this exercise until you feel emotionally peaceful and clear.

Exercise 16: Breathing in Forgiveness

It is not only important to release negative emotions and resentment, but also to forgive anyone who we feel has caused us pain and hurt. It is only with forgiveness that we are able to deeply hold love in our heart and genuinely express that love to others. This exercise uses breathing to help restore feelings of forgiveness and openness in our hearts.

- Lie flat on your back with your knees pulled up. Keep your feet slightly apart. Try to breathe in and out through your nose.

- Inhale deeply and begin to feel your heart soften. Begin to allow feelings of forgiveness and caring to fill your heart, your mind and every cell of your body. Feel yourself enveloped by feelings of love and understanding for anyone who you feel has hurt you. These feelings will bring a sense of peace and calm to your heart.

- Then exhale deeply and feel any negative emotions that may be lingering dissipate and wash away.

- Continue to repeat this exercise until you feel emotionally peaceful and clear.

Exercise 17: Love and Gratitude Meditation

This is a great meditation to do to help you reconnect with the healing power of love, forgiveness, and gratitude.

- Find a quiet spot where you can sit or lie comfortably.

- Close your eyes, and let your arms rest easily at your side. As you take a deep breath, focus on the area of your heart (located just to the left of the center of your chest).

- As you slowly inhale and exhale, imagine you're filling your heart with love. Feel the area surrounding your heart soften and expand as you fill it with loving and peaceful energy.

- Now, direct your breath into all of the parts of your body, starting with your feet and moving up through your body, finally into your head and neck.

- Notice any areas where you have stored any negative or upsetting emotions such as frustration, anger, or other feelings that make certain parts of your body feel tense, tight, heavy, or devitalized.

- Keep breathing love into those parts of your body until they, too, relax and soften. By the time you're done, you should feel much more quiet and peaceful.

- Now visualize your love radiating out from you and touching everyone you love and care about. If you choose to, you can send your love and the spirit of healing to your community, to our country, and even the entire earth.

- Now gently open your eyes and slowly begin to move around again. Enjoy the feelings of love, peace, and gratitude you have created.

Exercise 18: Loving Visualization

I want to share a loving visualization with you. It is meant to give you a few minutes to turn inward and get back in touch with loving yourself through self-nurturance. This will help you release any negative thoughts or upsets you may have accumulated throughout the day and help you reconnect with the healing power of love.

To do this visualization, find a quiet spot where you can sit or lie comfortably. As you take a deep breath, focus on the area of your heart (located just to the left of the center of your chest).

- As you inhale and exhale slowly and deeply, close your eyes and envision your heart as a luminous, emerald green jewel glowing with love and sending out brilliant light from behind your breastbone, where your heart resides.

- As you breathe slowly, begin to fill your heart with love. Feel the area surrounding your heart soften and expand as you fill it with loving and peaceful energy.

- Then, send love and appreciation to every part of your body, even the parts that you are concerned about or feel are less than lovable. They are all parts of you and worthy of the deepest love and caring.

- Breathe love and appreciation into your head, neck, shoulders, chest and down your arms and hands.

- Send this loving and healing breath next into your abdomen, hips, legs and feet.

- Continue loving and appreciating yourself until you feel your entire body overflowing with love.

- Now, gently open your eyes and slowly begin to move around again. Enjoy the feelings of love, peace and gratitude you have created.

Exercise 19: Divine Healing Water

- Sit or lie in a comfortable position, with your arms resting gently by your sides.

- Now, close your eyes and breathe deeply. Let your breathing be slow and relaxed.

- Visualize a river of living water flowing gently through you. This is Divine healing water, full of God's light and love.

- Feel this healing water flow into every cell of your body, cleansing you of all cares and worries, bringing you the deepest peace.

- Let this healing water flow through your head, renewing your mind and then moving into your neck and shoulders. As it moves through you, it carries away any tension and tightness.

- Then feel this Divine water flow gently into your chest and down your arms and hands, and then into your abdomen, bringing with it healing and life energy.

- Next, let this water move into your hips and pelvis and down into your legs and feet.

- As this Divine water leaves your body, all darkness is disappearing and is being replaced by light, love and happiness.

- Let this Divine healing water flow through you as long as you would like it to. Continue this process until you feel totally at peace and deeply relaxed.

Exercise 20: Breathing in the Divine Connection

As I mentioned in the introduction to this book, according to the Book of Genesis in the Old Testament, God created man from the dust of the earth and then breathed life into him. God continues to give us life every time that we take a breath. As such, breathing is literally a sacred act, one that connects us directly to our Creator.

In this exercise, you will be focusing on your connection to the Creator. Whenever I do this exercise slowly and peacefully, I feel a renewed sense of God's continual presence in my life. I am always filled with awe and wonder at the gift of life that God has given me.

- Lie flat on your back with your knees pulled up. Keep your feet slightly apart.

- Inhale deeply. As you breathe in, allow your stomach to relax so that the air flows into your abdomen. Let your stomach balloon out as you breathe in. Visualize the lowest parts of your lungs filling up with air.

- Now exhale deeply. As you breathe out, imagine the air being pushed out from the bottom of your lungs to the top.

- As you breathe in and out, feel God's love, caring and compassion surround you and fill every cell of your body. Know that you are a very precious to God and that God holds you close to His heart.

- Repeat this sequence until you feel a deep sense of peace and calm from knowing that you are totally loved and are a child of our Divine Creator.

Exercise 21: Divine Healing Breath

This is one of my favorite and most inspirational breathing and meditation exercises. I always feel uplifted when I do this exercise. It is a beautiful meditation on filling yourself with the Divine light and love of God. This meditation will also help you release any tension or negativity from your mind and fill you with wonderful feelings of peace and joy.

- Begin the meditation by finding a quiet place. It can be a peaceful room in your house or office or even a beautiful spot in your backyard. Then, sit or lie in a comfortable position, with your arms resting gently by your sides.

- Close your eyes and breathe deeply. Let your breathing be slow and relaxed. Visualize yourself as a flower in the sun, opening yourself to God's light and love. Feel this Divine light surrounding you and enfolding you, filling every cell of your body with love.

- As this light fills and nurtures you, you are being cleansed of all cares and worries. This Divine light is dispelling all darkness as it gently and lovingly restores you to a state of health and peace.

- Visualize this Divine light, bringing brightness and clarity into your mind, your head and then your neck and shoulders. As it moves through you, it carries away any tension and tightness.

- As you continue to breathe deeply and slowly, feel the warmth of this light as it moves into your chest and down your arms and hands, and then into your abdomen, bringing with it healing and protection.

- Next, let this Divine light move into your hips and pelvis and finally down into your legs and feet.

- Let this Divine light move through you as long as you would like it to. Continue this process until you feel totally at peace and relaxed.

- Know that God is always with you, caring for you and loving you always.

7

Engage in Regular Aerobic Exercise

Besides deep breathing exercises, I also recommend engaging in regular aerobic exercise like walking, swimming, dancing, bicycling and yoga. Aerobic exercise refers to any type of exercise that increases the amount of oxygen contained in the body.

With aerobic exercise, you receive the great benefit of combining deep, slow breathing with movement. Not only does it energize your body and elevate your mood, but aerobic exercise has great health benefits for your entire body!

Walking is my favorite type of aerobic exercise. I am an avid walker, and have been since medical school—I walk at a moderate pace, breathing slowly and deeply to maximize the health and relaxation benefits. Often I walk with friends or family members. I have regular walking partners who I get together with and always look forward to talking and sharing with them as we walk together.

I live in the San Francisco Bay Area and there is a lot of natural beauty here- the bay, the surrounding mountains, lots of local parks, gardens and walking trails. We always try to find new places to explore. I love to walk after work which helps to melt away the stress of my busy day. I also get to enjoy the beautiful natural surroundings of the area that I live in while receiving the fabulous health benefits of regular exercise, which is why I do it nearly every day. The days I am not able to get out, I can literally feel a subtle drop in my energy level, and my mood isn't as cheery and bright. Walking also helps to keep me flexible and has kept my weight virtually the same as when I was in medical school.

I like to combine walking with a stretching routine in which I also practice slow, deep breathing. Techniques that help to promote physical flexibility, such as stretching and yoga have a number of health benefits. Not only do they keep you supple and flexible flexibility, but these techniques also significantly enhance the mechanics of breathing. This assists in the flow of life giving oxygen to the cells while promoting the removal of carbon dioxide, one of our main waste products of metabolism.

These slow, methodical exercises also reduce muscle tension. As you relax, the other effects of stress are gradually reduced. Also, stretching exercises and yoga can be practiced almost anywhere, which is a great benefit to travelers.

My advice: I recommend that you engage in moderate, regular aerobic exercise at least three to five times a week for thirty to sixty minutes per session. Doing this on a regular basis will not only improve your physical and mental energy, but will also help to reduce the risk of heart attack, cancer, and depression as well as many other health problems. If you've been sedentary, start with 10 minutes a day and work your way up to 30 minutes to an hour a day. Whichever activity you select, you will be vastly improving your health and overall well-being.

A cautionary note: If your goal is to improve your level of oxygenation and expand your breathing capacity, I recommend that you avoid or limit doing high-intensity activities such as running, triathlons, competitive cycling, mountain climbing, tennis, and power walk.

While these strenuous types of exercises can feel very good in the short run, they are more anaerobic than aerobic and actually deplete the oxygen levels of the body. They are also more contractive and acidifying to the body. These types of exercises are more likely to deplete both the oxygen content and the natural buffering agents contained within the muscles, as well as to generate lactic acid. They actually contract your diaphragm and the muscles of your chest. This works against the health giving benefits of oxygenating your body through deep, slow breathing. This is especially important for women who are in their forties, fifties and older in whom maintaining healthy oxygen levels becomes more and more crucial to their physical, mental and emotional health and well-being.

Health Benefits of Aerobic Exercise

Muscles become energized and toned: When you participate in aerobic exercise, you create a pumping action of the muscles that helps to move oxygen, blood, and nutrients throughout the body. With regular aerobic exercise, skeletal muscles become energized and toned, making every movement, from lifting objects to walking, more easily accomplished. Exercise can help improve posture, which increases oxygenation through structural realignment.

Improves heart and lung health: This includes the muscles of the heart and lungs. As a result, aerobic exercise also conditions the heart and lungs to work more efficiently. As the heart becomes conditioned, it is able to pump more blood with each stroke. Thus, it can circulate the same volume of blood with fewer strokes and doesn't have to work as hard.

Once an exercise program is initiated, the resting heart rate soon slows down quite markedly. Research studies show that the beneficial changes can occur rapidly, often within several months. A lower resting heart rate means more than increased strength and stamina. A healthier heart also reacts less dramatically during episodes of anxiety and stress. When anxiety causes the adrenal glands to pump out stressor hormones, a conditioned heart will not experience a significant rise in the heart rate.

In a stressful situation, a fit person may have only a slight rise in heart rate, while a sedentary person may experience a terrifying pounding of the heart and shortness of breath. Not only does a fit woman tend to stay calmer and more in control of her emotions during a taxing situation, but in periods of extreme stress, her good physical conditioning may help prevent a heart attack and thereby save her life.

The lungs also benefit from aerobic exercise. Regular aerobic exercise helps us to breathe more deeply and efficiently, thereby improving oxygenation and nutrient flow to tissues throughout the entire body. With this type of exercise, you will tend to breathe more deeply and slowly. Over time, this helps to improve the elasticity of your lungs and relaxes the diaphragm and chest muscles, thereby allowing you to inhale more oxygen

It also aids in the removal of waste products such as carbon dioxide, lactic acid, and other products of metabolism through exhalation by the lungs. The acidity or pH of the blood is lowered to an optimal range and helps to create a state of slight alkalinity within our bodies which is ideal for cellular and tissue function and the efficient production of energy by the cells. This is important since optimal energy production is needed to run the body's many chemical and physiological functions.

Helps to discharge and relieve stress: The problem for many women who are feeling overwhelmed by chronic stress is that their sympathetic nervous system is always in a state of readiness to react to a perceived crisis. This puts them in a constant state of tension, causing them to react to small stresses the same way they react to real emergencies. Their adrenal glands increase their out-put of adrenaline and cortisone, and their thyroid gland pumps out thyroxin (the thyroid hormone), adjusting the body chemistry to meet the crisis. Their heart speeds up, their pulses race, and their neck and shoulder muscles tense, as do muscles in other parts of the body.

These tight and tense muscles have decreased blood flow and oxygenation. Waste products such as excessive carbon dioxide accumulate in this physical environment and can further worsen fight-or-flight symptoms. In addition, stress causes breathing to become rapid and shallow. Less oxygen is taken in through respiration, which further decreases the oxygen available to the muscles and internal organs.

The tension that accumulates in the body to meet this "emergency" must then be discharged. Often it is discharged emotionally by yelling at children or being irritable and abrupt with people at work. Some women just feel overwhelmed by the many responsibilities and details of life. Many of my women patients have shared with me that they deal with this fight-or-flight reaction by discharging their feeling of stress and anxiety through binging on junk food, alcohol, sugar or cigarette addictions. For example, overeating can become a way of diffusing tension. Unfortunately, the habitual indulgence in addictive behavior is harmful to the body.

Physical exercise, particularly aerobic, is a great antidote to relieving stress. It discharges the fight-or-flight tension without harming either your body or personal relationships and it helps to bring your nervous system back into a state of balance.

Supports healthy emotions: Regular aerobic exercise also promotes a balanced healthy mood. After exercising, you will feel more peaceful, calmer, and even happier. You will certainly feel more refreshed and energized. Research studies have also shown that regular aerobic exercise like walking also greatly reduces depression. In fact, walking has been found to be as effective as antidepressant medication in elevating mood in depressed individuals.

How does exercise promote such striking emotional changes? Exercise brings better oxygenation and circulation to the brain and nerves by opening up and dilating blood vessels of the head and brain. Thus, more nutrients can flow into and more waste products can be removed from this vital system. In fact, 20 percent of the blood flow from the heart goes directly to the brain. The brain also utilizes a large share (again, 20 percent) of the body's nutrients and energy.

Supports healthy brain function: Research studies done on adults who do regular aerobic exercise compared with similar groups who are sedentary show striking differences in a variety of mental functions. Adults engaged in an active exercise program were shown to have better concentration, and clearer and quicker thinking and better problem solving capability. In addition, reaction time and short-term memory improved. This can be an important preventive benefit for women past midlife who want to preserve peak intellectual and mental capacity for the rest of their lives.

Helps to relieve symptoms of female health issues: Not only does regular exercise induce functional improvements in the brain, it also dramatically alters brain chemistry in a positive way through the increased production of beta endorphins. Beta endorphins, chemicals released from the pituitary glands, act as natural opiates. They are chemically similar to the pain reliever morphine, but 200 times more potent.

Endorphins have a dramatic effect on mood. When levels in the body are high, they improve a woman's general sense of well-being. Beta endorphin levels increase after ovulation, during the early part of the second half of the menstrual cycle (called luteal phase by physicians). As menstruation approaches, beta endorphin levels can begin to fall. In fact, some PMS researchers believe that the drop in beta endorphins may be responsible for the emotional symptoms of PMS such as anxiety, irritability, and mood swings. These are the predominant symptoms in more than 80 percent of women with PMS.

Exercise helps reduce anxiety and nervous tension by increasing the production of beta endorphins. Measurements of beta endorphins taken a half hour after the exercise session have shown that beta endorphin levels were still higher than at starting. Some women who exercise regularly report related feelings of elation, euphoria, and even bliss. Aerobic exercise may even help cushion the premenstrual fall in beta endorphins and thereby reduce PMS-related anxiety.

Research studies have also shown that regular aerobic exercise also decreases the risk of endometriosis and reduces menstrual cramps and pain. It also significantly reduces the incidence of hot flashes of women in menopause and helps to promote deeper, sounder sleep. This is a great benefit for many women in menopause who suffer from sleeplessness or insomnia.

Regular aerobic exercise also supports bone and heart health, sex drive or libido, memory and cognitive function and reduces weight gain in postmenopausal women. It also significantly helps to reduce the risk of breast cancer. The circulatory and oxygenation benefits of regular aerobic exercise support the health of all your organs, including the uterus and ovaries.

Improves metabolic function: Regular aerobic exercise helps to stabilize hypoglycemia and reduce the roller coaster effect that it has on the mood and body. It also protects again diabetes by creating a decrease in total glucose and insulin. It also helps to reduce risk factors of heart disease by increasing HDL ("good") cholesterol promoting a decrease in triglycerides. Women who engage in the deep healthy breathing and skeletal muscle movement of regular walking also have a decrease in mid-thigh fat and an increase in mid thigh muscle.

For women who are concerned about their weight, it reduces excessive cravings for food, both for women with food addictions and for women with PMS who tend to overeat high-stress foods in the week or two prior to the onset of menstruation. This curbing of excessive appetite and over-eating improves our ability to lose and maintain weight. Exercise also improves the body's ability to burn calories more efficiently and rapidly. This provides an additional boost to weight loss.

A regular exercise program also aids your appearance by helping preserve attractive body contours, toning muscles and improving skin condition. Exercise increases blood circulation to the skin, keeping the skin pink, soft, and supple. The skin of women who don't exercise frequently looks pale and unhealthy.

Exercise benefits the general health of many other systems, too. Elimination through the bowels and kidneys is improved, which also helps to regulate weight and water balance. Constipation is less likely to be a problem in active women. It reduces the tendency to anxiety-related digestive symptoms such as abdominal discomfort and bloating. In fact, I have had patients with stress-related intestinal symptoms report symptom relief immediately following exercise sessions. Exercise also helps reduce blood pressure levels, which takes stress off the heart and contributes to a reduction of heart attack risk. In summary, exercise benefits the entire body and promotes good health.

Increases the overall energy of the body: With aerobic exercise, the production of energy by the cells in the form of ATP also becomes more efficient. This is very beneficial since optimal energy production is needed to run the body's many chemical and physiological functions. In contrast, sedentary women have much less energy production and are prone to fatigue and tiredness.

Benefits of Exercise

Improves resistance to and relief of anxiety episodes

- Reduces the fight-or-flight response
- Promotes cardiovascular resistance to stress
- Decreases skeletal muscle tension
- Reduces pent-up aggression and frustration
- Promotes a feeling of calm and peace

Improves brain function

- Promotes better oxygenation and blood circulation to the brain
- Increases output of beta endorphins
- Improves concentration, problem solving, reaction time, and short-term memory

Improves psychological functions

- Decreases anxiety and nervous tension
- Produces a sense of well-being and even elation
- Reduces depression
- Reduces insomnia
- Improves sense of mastery and self-confidence
- Promotes development of beneficial habits
- Helps decrease harmful addictive behavior

Improves physiological functions

- Stabilizes blood sugar level
- Reduces food craving
- Helps weight loss and maintenance
- Improves elimination through the bowels and kidneys
- Improves digestive functions
- Reduces blood pressure

Before You Start, Be Prepared

As you can see, the power of exercise is far reaching—from helping to alleviate PMS and prevent breast cancer to easing hot flashes and decreasing your risk for heart attack—there isn't a system in your body that doesn't rejuvenate itself with regular exercise.

However, launching headfirst into a vigorous exercise regimen without giving your body an opportunity to adapt to this new routine is a setup for failure.

Exercise should be a lifestyle change, not a weekend romp. If you start slowly, include proper hydration, and treat injuries quickly and correctly, you'll be more likely to not just adopt a new exercise routine, but also stick with it.

Warm Up and Cool Down

The two most critical aspects of any exercise routine are what you do immediately before and after your actual workout. The "warm up" involves coaxing your body from a state of inactivity to one of motion. Warming up gets your body in gear; helping all your systems get ready for exercise.

To warm up, walk around gently swinging your arms and raising your knees. Gently stretch the muscles of your calves, the backs of your legs, your waist and back. Hold each stretching position for 30 to 45 seconds. Go to the point of tension but not pain; breathe deeply; and pay special attention to those parts of your body you will be exercising.

When you have finished your exercise, simply repeat this process to cool down.

Drink Enough Water

The need to keep your body well hydrated before, during, and after exercise is critical. Especially when you consider that we all consist mainly of water—water makes up 82 percent of blood, 75 percent of muscle, 25 percent of bone, 76 percent of brain tissue, and 90 percent of lung tissue!

Everything in your body depends on water, and when you exercise, you lose it through your sweat, breath, and urine. Moderate exercise in a temperate climate results in the loss of half a gallon of water per day, while heavy training can leave you two gallons drier each day.

When you are exercising, be sure to drink water throughout your workout. And remember, this is in addition to the eight glasses you need each day for normal, healthy functioning.

Finally, if you are an estrogen deficient-fast processor, you may find it useful to take moderate amounts of sodium bicarbonate (baking soda) before, during, and after exercising to reduce and even prevent stiffness and sore muscles. Just drinking one-half to one teaspoon of baking soda dissolved in an 8-ounce glass of distilled water will do the trick.

To summarize, I want to ensure that you are most successful in starting and maintaining a regular aerobic exercise program. Be sure to start slowly, include proper hydration, and treat injuries quickly and correctly. That way, you'll be more likely to not just adopt a new exercise routine, but also stick with it.

Stay Injury-Free

The following tips will prime your body for peak performance, and help to keep you injury-free.

Invest in a good pair of comfortable shoes, such as Ryka—a wonderful brand of shoes made just for women. I like their shoes because they are designed to take into account a woman's narrower heels and wider forefoot. Ryka can be found in most Lady Foot Locker stores or ordered online at ryka.com. Whichever brand you choose, make sure your sneakers offer plenty of support and cushioning. And to prevent ankle or foot injury, replace your shoes when you notice the heels wearing down—at least every four to six months.

Exercise outside if weather allows. Take time to rejoice in nature and the change of the seasons. If the weather doesn't allow for outside activity, move your routine to a nearby mall or try the treadmill at a nearby gym.

Continue to challenge yourself and add variety to your routine. If you start off walking for 10 to 15 minutes a day three days a week, try building to 20 to 30 minutes a day, then try to walk four or five days a week. Ideally, you should work towards a goal of walking for one hour a day, six to seven days a week.

Finally, **build a community around exercise.** Find a walking partner or join a walking club. It is easy to find excuses for not taking your morning walk, but those excuses won't hold up if someone is waiting for you on the corner or at the gym.

Combatting Health Conditions that Can Prevent You From Exercising

As wonderful as aerobic activity is, I know how difficult it can be to move even one step when faced with pain and discomfort. While it seems like rest would be your best bet, the truth is exercise almost always accelerates healing. Whether you have a short-term or lifelong condition, I encourage you to find creative ways to adapt your exercise program so you can still get the health benefits, without stressing the parts of your body that need special consideration.

Here are some of the most common roadblocks that can stand in the way of lacing up those shoes, and helpful strategies on how to get around them.

Excess Weight

Obesity is an epidemic in this country, and exercise is the absolute best way to cure it. However, walking can be a challenge for women who are extremely overweight. A study published in the *Journal of Applied Physiology* found that one in four obese patients who started taking brisk daily walks suffered knee injuries, and one in four of those injured patients never returned to exercise, suggesting that walking is bad for your knees if you're overweight.

However, the walkers in this study covered more ground-2½ feet or more per stride—which significantly increases knee strain, especially if body weight is excessive. The same study concluded that when taking shorter strides, which allow for carrying on a normal conversation without getting winded, even obese walkers had no significant increase in risk of knee injury.

If you're overweight, take shorter strides and walk at a slow, steady pace. Just don't give up—as the pounds melt off and your overall condition improves, your joints will become healthier and have less weight to carry. Then you can pick up the pace, if desired.

Knee Problems

The knees are the most commonly injured joints in the body, partly because the bones are secured by ligaments designed to hold them in position only when the knee is not under load. The bulky muscles around the knees—particularly the quadriceps (front of the thighs) and the hamstrings (back of the thighs)—are supposed to do the heavy work. But many women use those muscles only to propel themselves forward—and otherwise allow their quads and hamstrings to be passive, relying heavily on the ligaments.

Building up your quads and hamstring muscles and keeping them active are the best ways to protect your knees. If you have knee problems, I recommend consulting with a physician before starting any fitness routine. And, to avoid damaging the cushion under the kneecap, be sure to step lightly when walking—don't pound your feet into the ground, especially when walking downhill.

Osteoarthritis of the Hip

For most women with this very common condition, walking is the last thing on their agenda. But if you have some cartilage left in your hips, arthritis is usually a good reason to engage in regular aerobic exercise. That's because joint cartilage—the hardest-working part of your joints—has no direct blood supply of its own. Instead, like a sponge, it soaks in nutrient-rich joint fluid and cleans itself by discharging wastes into that same fluid, which is constantly replacing itself.

Weight-bearing exercise compresses your cartilage, causing the joint fluid to squeeze out. And when you release the weight, the cartilage expands and soaks up fresh fluid. In other words, walking stimulates your joints' circulatory system. Without exercise, the cartilage gets very little nutrition and becomes increasingly gritty with accumulated wastes.

So, with your physician's guidance, using a cane or walker if needed, start a walking routine at whatever level is appropriate for your condition. Even if you can only make one loop around a room, you'll be helping your hips immeasurably. Then gradually increase your frequency and duration at a pace that's comfortable.

Plantar Fasciitis

Plantar fasciitis, inflammation in the tissue connecting the heel bone to the toes, is the result of carrying your weight without proper foot support. It is often caused by chronic small tears that keep reoccurring due to overuse. It usually manifests as pain in the heel, especially after extended periods of rest, such as what you are experiencing first thing in the morning. Common culprits include spending all day on your feet and wearing high heels, which can triple the strain on those tissues.

If you continue to overstress this area, the repeated inflammation can result in new bone growth on the heel, often referred to as a heel spur. If you strongly suspect that this may be your problem, I recommend that you consult with a podiatrist who can examine your feet properly.

In the meantime, to get relief from plantar fasciitis, I recommend relaxing your feet with a 15-minute alkaline soak each evening. Make the soak by dissolving two or three teaspoons of baking soda in about 5 inches of warm water, in a dishpan-sized container. After soaking your feet, massage them for at least five minutes each by rolling them over a tennis ball.

And, as hard as it may be for some high-heel addicts, I recommend limiting the heel height of your shoes to two inches or less. Better yet, wear flat shoes. In addition, buy shoes in the evening, when feet are naturally a bit larger, and don't wear the same shoes all the time—this relentlessly stresses the same areas of the plantar fascia.

8

Nutritional Supplements that Improve Oxygenation

Research studies have found that a number of nutrients work synergistically with oxygen to support your health and wellness. These nutrients include several herbs which help to improve the health of the lungs and immune function in individuals with respiratory infections such as colds and flus and vasodilators, which promote good blood flow and healthy oxygenation of all our cells and tissues

Other nutritional supplements help to increase energy production within the body. Finally, some individuals, such as menstruating women with iron-deficiency anemia and athletes participating in anaerobic or endurance sports, may need other nutrients such as iron or sodium phosphate. Iron is necessary to insure the transport of sufficient oxygen by the red blood cells, while sodium phosphate assists in the release of oxygen from the red blood cells into the muscles.

Herbs That Improve the Health of the Lungs and Immune Function

Several different herbs support the health of the lungs as well as improve the immune function of the body.

Echinacea

Echinacea root has long been used in traditional botanical medicine for its immunity-enhancing properties. In recent years, a number of studies have confirmed the beneficial effects that echinacea has on immune response, particularly against respiratory conditions like colds and flus.

Research studies have found that using echinacea increases phagocytosis (the process by which cells of the immune system engulf and destroy pathogenic organisms), activates macrophages to destroy pathogenic organisms, and stimulates both T lymphocytes and B lymphocytes.

In a review article published in the *European Journal of Herbal Medicine*, the author summarized the findings of six clinical trials using echinacea for the treatment of colds and flus as well as six trials that evaluated echinacea for its preventive benefits. The results of these trials confirmed that echinacea improves immune function when used for the treatment of respiratory infections.

Suggested Dosage: Take two capsules three times per day (125 mg capsules that have been standardized to 3.2 percent to 4.8 percent echinacosides), or take ten to thirty drops of liquid extract three times per day standardized for 1 percent echinacosides.

Ginseng

Ginseng root has been used as a tonic to improve resistance to disease in Traditional Chinese Medicine for several thousand years. Research studies have confirmed that ginseng root improves immune function by stimulating the activity of natural killer cells and increasing the production of lymphocytes.

An article published in *Drugs Under Experimental and Clinical Research* discussed the results of a study in which the ability of ginseng to improve immune response to the influenza vaccine was evaluated versus a placebo. Two hundred twenty-seven adult volunteers were given either 100 mg of a standardized extract of ginseng root or a placebo daily over a twelve-week period. All of the volunteers were given an influenza vaccine at week four. The volunteers taking the ginseng root showed a significantly greater immune response to the influenza vaccine than did the placebo group. In addition, the individuals in the treatment group experienced fewer cases of influenza and fewer colds than those in the placebo group.

Suggested Dosage: For maximum benefit, take a high-quality preparation, an extract of the main root of a plant that is four to six years old, standardized for ginsenoside content and ratio. Twice a day, take a 100 mg capsule. If this is too stimulating, especially before bedtime, take the second dose midafternoon, or take only the morning dose.

Bromelain

Nasal congestion due to respiratory-tract infections is a nuisance, hampering almost any activity. There is scientific evidence that bromelain can be very useful in the treatment of upper-respiratory problems that generate mucus. Bromelain decreases the volume and viscosity of mucus so that it can be more easily cleared from the respiratory tract.

This was demonstrated in a study appearing in *Drugs Under Experimental and Clinical Research*. Volunteers included seventy men and fifty-four women, aged thirty-five to seventy-five, hospitalized with lung diseases such as chronic bronchitis, pneumonia, and pulmonary abscess. Patients were randomly given one of three therapies: amoxycillin plus 80 mg of bromelain, amoxycillin plus indomethacin, or amoxycillin alone, every eight hours, for at least eight days or as needed. The sputum (substance expelled by coughing or clearing the throat) of the patients was then analyzed for viscosity.

The results of this study showed that bromelain significantly increased the fluidity of mucus. There was also evidence that bromelain combined with drug therapy enhanced the absorption of the amoxycillin.

Suggested Dosage: 500 to 1000 mg four to six times per day. Take both with and apart from meals.

Using bromelain with antibiotics. Several studies in the scientific literature document the effectiveness of bromelain in enhancing the action of antibiotics. In one research study, published in Experimental Medicine & Surgery, fifty-three hospitalized patients were given combined antibiotic and bromelain therapy to treat such potentially life-threatening diseases as pneumonia, bronchitis, thrombophlebitis, pyelonephritis, and rectal abscesses. Twenty-three of these patients had been unsuccessfully treated with antibiotic therapy alone. Of these, twenty-two responded favorably to the combined therapy.

Researchers also compared the length of stay for patients taking antibiotics alone or the combined therapy. Patients with pneumonia or bronchitis who were treated with antibiotics alone remained in the hospital for an average of ten days, as compared with those who also received enzyme therapy, who were able to leave the hospital after only six days.

Another study, published in the journal *Headache*, looked at the use of bromelain in combination with antibiotics for the treatment of acute sinusitis. Forty-eight patients were placed on standard therapy, which included antihistamines and analgesic agents, along with antibiotics, if indicated. Twenty-three patients received bromelain four times daily, while the remaining twenty-five received a placebo. Of the patients receiving bromelain, 87 percent had complete resolution of nasal mucosal inflammation, compared with only 52 percent in the placebo group.

The next time you come down with an acute respiratory infection and your doctor writes you a prescription for antibiotics; consider supplementing that medication with bromelain. Along with rest, supplementing with bromelain will help you return to your usual activities much more quickly.

Vasodilators That Improve Oxygenation

Several substances called vasodilators promote greatly improved oxygenation of all the cells and tissues of the body. Unlike oxygen therapies, which actually supplement the level of oxygen contained within the body, these substances act, in part, to improve circulation. As a result, oxygen is better able to reach areas of the body that have been devitalized either by poor circulation due to hardening of the arteries, or by vasoconstriction (narrowing of the blood vessels) due to stress, cold, or other environmental factors, hormonal imbalances, or disease. These substances include gingko biloba, a powerful circulation-enhancing herb and l-arginine which stimulate the production of nitric oxide, a potent vasodilator produced within our bodies.

Gingko biloba

The ginkgo biloba tree species originated about 250 million years ago, and a single tree can live as long as 1000 years. This handsome tree is often planted in urban settings, as it resists disease, insects, and pollution. Modern science is finding that this ancient plant can also help slow the aging of the brain, alleviate depression, and, perhaps most importantly, improve circulation and oxygenation throughout the body. Ginkgo leaf extracts are used by individuals throughout the world for their circulatory and oxygenation benefits.

The chemicals found in ginkgo have powerful vasodilating effects: They act by stimulating the release of prostacyclin (a prostaglandin hormone) and a vascular relaxing substance. These chemicals also improve the tone of blood vessels and reduce the stickiness of red blood cells, so that they flow more smoothly through the blood vessels as they carry oxygen throughout the body.

Numerous research studies confirm the benefits of ginkgo extracts on all parts of the circulatory system, improving blood flow and oxygenation to the brain, heart, and other vital organs and the extremities. It is useful for many conditions including coronary-artery disease, cerebral vascular insufficiency, peripheral vascular disease, Alzheimer's disease, Reynaud's disease (vasoconstriction of the extremities), impotence due to diminished blood flow, diseases of the eye due to diabetes mellitus or poor circulation, cyclic edema due to PMS, and even clinical depression (gingko acts as a potent mood elevator).

Many important performance traits are enhanced by the improvement in the oxygenation of the body that occurs when using ginkgo. These include improvements in physical energy, mental clarity, cognitive function, mood, and ability to socialize. Side effects are rare; however, women should be aware that the flavonoid quercetin, which is found in ginkgo, may lower estrogen production within the body.

Suggested Dosage: Only standardized extracts should be used (standardized to 24 percent flavonoid glycosides and 6 percent terpene lactones). Dosages may vary between 40 to 60 mg, two to three times a day.

L-Arginine

L-arginine is a powerful supplement which supports the production of nitric oxide within our bodies. Nitric oxide is a substance produced by our bodies that helps to optimize the flow of blood through the arteries and veins. As a potent vasodilator, it enhances the flow of blood and the transport of oxygen to all the cells and tissues of the body. Research studies suggest that nitric oxide may actually be one of the most important chemicals that our bodies produce.

Nitric oxide is a gaseous molecule produced in the body from the amino acid arginine. Extensive research shows that nitric oxide is involved in regulating a wide variety of physiologic functions. In fact, some of these studies suggest that nitric oxide may even increase the level of oxygen within the body. For example, in patients with chronic lung diseases such as chronic obtrusive lung disease and adult respiratory distress syndrome, inhalation of nitric oxide improved oxygenation.

Insufficient levels of nitric oxide are associated with many disease conditions, most of which relate to poor circulation and insufficient oxygenation. These include diseases of the heart and lungs and of the neuroendocrine, immune, reproductive, and other systems. Insufficient nitric oxide production can also greatly hamper one's level of performance in many important areas of life, leading to diminished physical and mental energy and immune function, erectile dysfunction (in men), diminished sexual responsiveness (in women), poor recovery from exertion and injury, and impaired wound healing.

Nitric oxide production enhances sports performance in activities such as body building, football, swimming, and bicycle riding, where good muscular development and healthy circulation provide a competitive edge. It is also known that levels of nitric oxide tend to decrease with age.

Not only does optimal production of nitric oxide increase performance capability, but it also contributes to the "look of success" that many peak performers have, because it enhances peripheral circulation. High nitric oxide producers typically have healthy skin and hair, and well-developed muscles. In contrast, elderly individuals (and even younger individuals with diminished nitric oxide production) often have thinner hair and paler, thinner skin.

Nitric oxide production levels can be increased through nutritional supplementation with l-arginine, a semi-essential amino acid, thereby improving vasodilation and oxygenation. This can greatly improve both health and performance capability. Research studies have shown that intravenous administration of the amino acid l-arginine can increase nitric oxide production in humans. L-arginine can also be taken as a nutritional supplement.

Suggested Dosage: Up to six grams per day may be taken. Its use should be avoided in individuals with a history of recent heart attack, pregnant women with pre-eclampsia, recurrent herpes infections, severe allergies or asthma.

Nutrients That Improve Energy Production

The following nutrients are utilized in combination with oxygen within our bodies for optimal energy production. Along with deep, slow breathing techniques, I highly recommend the use of these nutrients, including coenzyme Q-10, magnesium, potassium, and vitamin B complex. This is especially important for individuals who are in their forties and beyond and want to maintain or improve their physical and mental energy or even to improve cardiovascular function. Except for coenzyme Q-1-0, younger women in their twenties and thirties who have busy, strenuous lives can greatly benefit from these nutrients, also.

Coenzyme Q-10

Along with oxygen, coenzyme Q-10 helps to maximize the amount of energy that can be produced within the body as adenosine triphosphate (ATP), the main energy currency of the body. Coenzyme Q-10 belongs to a family of brightly colored substances called quinones, which occur widely in nature. Good dietary sources of coenzyme Q-10 include whole grains, fish, organ meats, soybean oil, walnuts, and sesame seeds.

It is also produced within our bodies, where it acts as an electron carrier in the energy cycles that take place within the cell that lead to the production of ATP. It is a powerful antioxidant. Coenzyme Q-10 works in conjunction with vitamin E to scavenge free radicals, thereby protecting the tissues of the body from oxidative damage.

Unfortunately, our production of coenzyme Q-10 diminishes with age, which can have a limiting effect on the amount of energy we are able to produce. Many individuals who are middle-aged and older can benefit from the use of supplemental coenzyme Q-10. Not only does it increase the level of energy production within the body, but it has also been found to act as a mild metabolic stimulant.

Research studies have also found that it improves cardiac function. Its usefulness in treating individuals with heart failure is probably due to its ability to improve energy production within the heart muscle cells. Coenzyme Q-10 has been found to enhance both the pumping and electrical functions of the heart.

It is also used by some endurance athletes who often have an increased need for coenzyme Q-10, as well as individuals on anti-aging programs.

Suggested Dosage: The dosage of coenzyme Q-10 ranges from 50 to 100 mg a day. Physicians may recommend that patients with specific health conditions take even higher dosages. Other antioxidants—such as vitamin E, vitamin C, vitamin A (as beta-carotene), selenium, and zinc—should be used in conjunction with coenzyme Q-10.

Magnesium

The body requires adequate levels of magnesium in order to maintain energy and vitality. The process of aerobic metabolism requires magnesium to produce ATP. When magnesium is deficient, ATP production falls and the body forms lactic acid. Accumulation of lactic acid can lead to acidosis and a drop in energy levels. Therefore, having sufficient amounts of magnesium helps to maintain a high level of physical energy.

This has been confirmed in a number of research studies. For example, a study reported at a conference on magnesium described that when 200 individuals were given magnesium supplements, 198 of them experienced relief from fatigue, a remarkably high result.

Suggested Dosage: Magnesium is given in divided doses, 400 to 1000 mg daily. There is a possible laxative effect at higher dosages. It is important to maintain a healthy calcium to magnesium ratio. Optimal levels are considered to be in a 2:1 or 10:4 ratio with calcium predominating over magnesium.

Potassium

Like magnesium, potassium has a powerful enhancing effect on energy and vitality. Potassium deficiency has been associated with fatigue and muscular weakness. One form of potassium, in particular — called potassium aspartate — has been found to be particularly useful for restoring the level of energy in individuals with chronic fatigue. It has been combined with magnesium aspartate in a number of clinical studies on fatigue.

Aspartic acid plays a vital role in aerobic (oxygen-dependent) energy production within the cells and helps transport both potassium and magnesium into the cells. Potassium aspartate has been shown in a number of clinical trials to reduce fatigue after five or six weeks of constant use. Even within ten days, many volunteers began to feel better. The benefits of potassium were seen in 90 percent of the people tested. Magnesium aspartate also has the same effects.

Suggested Dosage: The recommended dosage for potassium and/or potassium aspartate is 100 to 300 mg per day. Potassium supplements can cause intestinal irritation in susceptible individuals, particularly those with preexisting intestinal disease.

Vitamin B-Complex

Vitamin B complex consists of a group of eleven separate nutrients: thiamine, riboflavin, niacin, pantothenic acid, pyridoxine (vitamin B6), folic acid, biotin, para-aminobenzoic acid (PABA), vitamin B12, choline, and inositol. In many cases they participate in the same chemical reactions in the body; therefore, they need to be taken together for best results. The B vitamins play a critical role in the conversion of carbohydrates into energy. When carbohydrates are "burned" within the cells in the presence of oxygen, much more energy is released to fuel the needs of the body than can be produced in the absence of oxygen. Various B vitamins are necessary for this conversion to progress efficiently.

Suggested Dosage: B-complex vitamins may be taken in a dosage of 25 to 100 mg a day, as a single dose or in divided dosages. It is best to take the B vitamins during the day, rather than at night, as they can be stimulating and can cause some people to have difficulty falling asleep.

Nutrients That Support Oxygen-Carrying Capability and pH Balance

Several nutrients are needed to promote the healthy functioning of red blood cells. Red blood cells carry oxygen to the cells and tissues throughout the body.

Iron

Iron is an important mineral that exists in the body in combination with protein. In the bloodstream, iron combines with copper and protein to form hemoglobin, which provides the coloration of the red blood cell. Hemoglobin binds with oxygen, enabling it to be transported from the lungs to all the cells of the body via the circulation.

Iron is also used by the body to produce myoglobin, which is found in muscle tissue. Myoglobin also acts as a transporter of oxygen, but only to muscle cells. Since oxygen plays such an important role in the production of energy within the cells, iron is needed in sufficient amounts if one is to have the physical and mental energy necessary for peak performance.

Women are at particular risk of iron-deficiency anemia because of menstruation. Anemia is associated with a diminished capacity to do physical activity, due, in part, to poor oxygenation. In a controlled study published in the *American Journal of Clinical Nutrition*, seventy-five women were given a treadmill test. Those with the most severe iron-deficiency anemia were able to stay on the treadmill an average of eight minutes less than the women without anemia. Further, none of the anemic women were able to perform under the highest workload conditions, while all of the women with adequate iron levels could.

Some athletes, both males and females, have been found to have low iron stores, despite normal blood profiles. Low iron stores can significantly affect athletic performance. Athletes tend to be at higher risk of iron deficiency than the rest of the population for several reasons. Iron is lost through perspiration while performing physically demanding exercise. Physically demanding exercise can also cause hemolysis or the breaking apart of blood cells. Iron lost from the blood cells through hemolysis is excreted from the body. In addition, acidosis and small amounts of intestinal bleeding can occur during heavy training, further depleting the body's store of iron.

Suggested Dosage: Dosage depends on gender and age. An average dosage is 15 mg per day, but a menstruating woman who is anemic may need as much as 30 to 70 mg a day until her iron reserves have been restored and her blood count has returned to normal.

Athletes who are engaged in heavy training may need as much as 25 mg of supplemental iron each day to maintain their reserves. Other supplemental nutrients such as folic acid, vitamin B12, vitamin B6, vitamin E, vitamin C, and zinc may also be necessary to restore and maintain a healthy blood profile in anemic individuals.

Postmenopausal women who are no longer menstruating have reduced requirements for iron supplementation. Research studies have indicated that high levels of iron are associated with an increased risk of heart disease in men.

Phosphorus (sodium phosphate)

Iron is not the only mineral necessary for the healthy functioning of red blood cells. Phosphorus is needed for the production of an enzyme called 2, 3-diphosphoglycerate (2, 3-DPG), which is found in red blood cells. Red blood cells transport oxygen in the blood to the tissues; 2, 3-DPG insures that oxygen, an important alkalinizing agent, is delivered to the muscles. It reduces the affinity that hemoglobin has for oxygen, so oxygen is more available to the tissues. Along with oxygen, phosphorus also promotes energy production within the cells. It also improves the production and use of glycogen, a sugar that is a ready source of energy in the muscles.

Because the typical American diet contains plentiful amounts of meat and dairy products, which contain large amounts of phosphorus, most people are far from deficient. However, athletes may need particularly high amounts of this mineral, since research studies have shown that muscles lose phosphorus into the bloodstream during periods of intense physical effort. The more a person exercises, the more phosphorus is needed by the body. Endurance athletes such as marathon runners will have low levels of phosphorus immediately after participating in an athletic event. Loss of phosphorus can impair buffering within the muscle tissue and limit the amount of oxygen delivered to the muscle cells.

Suggested Dosage: Phosphorus is given to athletes in a buffered form as sodium phosphate. It is used as an aid to improve sports performance. A typical dosage is 4 g a day, taken for three days prior to participating in an event. This has been found to improve both anaerobic and endurance performance. Sodium phosphate is nontoxic in normal amounts. However, taking large doses can lead to calcium loss, as phosphorus interacts with calcium metabolism.

9

Eat a Diet High in Oxygen

If you wish to follow a diet to help support and maintain the level of oxygen within your body then it is important to follow an alkaline, mostly vegetarian diet. As I've discussed throughout this book, oxygen is one of the most energy-enhancing and alkalinizing substances within our bodies.

It is best maintained by eating lots of raw, fresh fruits (except citrus fruits and berries, which tend to be highly acidic), vegetables, sprouted seeds, grains, beans, and green-food supplements such as spirulina, chlorella, wheat grass, and barley grass. These foods should be eaten in concert with other high-nutrient foods, some of which may require cooking, such as starches, whole grains, legumes, seeds and nuts, fish, and free-range poultry.

Fresh fruits and vegetables, in particular, tend to be high in oxygen content. This is because they are largely composed of water, which is made up of hydrogen and oxygen, and is mostly oxygen by weight. These foods are also excellent sources of alkaline minerals such as magnesium and potassium, which are needed, along with adequate oxygen, for the production of energy within our cells. They are also rich in antioxidants such as beta-carotene and vitamin C, which protect our cells from free-radical damage.

In contrast, a highly acidic diet will make you more prone to oxygen-depleting acidosis. These include foods high in refined sugar, saturated fat, and animal protein, such as red meat and dairy products. Stimulants, such as caffeine found in coffee, black tea, and cola drinks (which are also acidic), can provide a rapid pick-me-up, but this is often followed by a drop in energy. This is because these foods destabilize our blood sugar level as well as stress the adrenal glands.

These kinds of foods will reduce the level of energy, deplete the stores of oxygen, and increase the level of acidic waste products within the body. The only individuals who can tolerate a highly acidic diet are naturally strong oxygenators who have exceptional lung capacity or people who are very alkaline in constitution.

In addition, you should avoid food that is heavily processed, fried, boiled, or breaded, this type of preparation either causes food to lose essential energy-enhancing nutrients or produces free radicals in the cooking process, thereby increasing oxidative stress in the body. Lightly steamed food is preferable, as more essential nutrients are retained.

Following a diet that helps to maintain high levels of oxygen in the body is absolutely crucial to good health and peak performance. Many people notice a significant increase in their level of energy and zest for life when switching from an oxygen-depleting, highly acidic diet to an oxygen-enhancing, mostly vegetarian diet. In addition, there's usually a significant improvement in health, as colds, flus, aches and pains, indigestion, and fatigue begin to diminish.

About Susan M. Lark, M.D.

Dr. Susan Lark is one of the foremost authorities in the fields of women's health care and alternative medicine. Dr. Lark has successfully treated many thousands of women emphasizing holistic health and complementary medicine in her clinical practice. Her mission is to provide women with unique, safe and effective alternative therapies to greatly enhance their health and well-being.

A graduate of Northwestern University Feinberg School of Medicine, she has served on the clinical faculty of Stanford University Medical School, and taught in their Division of Family and Community Medicine.

Dr. Lark is a distinguished clinician, author, lecturer and innovative product developer. Through her extensive clinical experience, she has been an innovator in the use of self-care treatments such as diet, nutrition, exercise and stress management techniques in the field of women's health, and has lectured extensively throughout the United States on topics in preventive medicine. She is the author of many best-selling books on women's health. Her signature line of nutritional supplements and skin care products are available through healthydirections.com.

One of the most widely referenced physicians on the Internet, Dr. Lark has appeared on numerous radio and television shows, and has been featured in magazines and newspapers including: Real Simple, Reader's Digest, McCall's, Better Homes & Gardens, New Woman, Mademoiselle, Harper's Bazaar, Redbook, Family Circle, Seventeen, Shape, Great Life, The New York Times, The Chicago Tribune, and The San Francisco Chronicle.

She has also served as a consultant to major corporations, including the Kellogg Company and Weider Nutrition International, and was spokesperson for The Gillette Company Women's Cancer Connection.

Dr. Lark can be contacted at (650) 561-9978 to make an appointment for a consultation.

We would enjoy hearing from you! Please share your success stories, requests for new topics and comments with us. Our team at Dr. Susan's Healthy Living may be contacted at drsusanshealthyliving@gmail.com. We invite you to visit our website for Dr. Lark's newest books at drsusanshealthyliving.com.

NOTES

NOTES

www.ingramcontent.com/pod-product-compliance
Lightning Source LLC
Chambersburg PA
CBHW080054280326
41934CB00014B/3312